Thank you, Nurse!

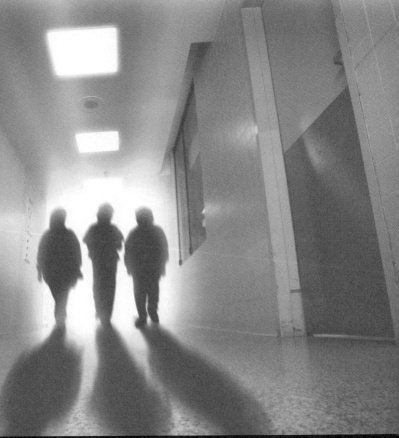

Debbie Phillips, R.N.
with Ned Carnes

THANK YOU,
NURSE!

Inquiries regarding permission for use of the material contained in this book should be addressed to:

> CornerStone Leadership Institute
> P.O. Box 764087
> Dallas, TX 75376
> 888.789.LEAD

Printed in the United States of America
ISBN-13: 978-0-9798009-0-0
ISBN-10: 0-9798009-0-0

Credits

Design, art direction, and production	Melissa Monogue, Back Porch Creative, Plano, TX info@BackPorchCreative.com
Copy Editor	Kathleen Green, Positively Proofed, Plano, TX info@PositivelyProofed.com

CONTENTS

INTRODUCTION

> "Trained nurses, whose gentle ministrations in the sick-room,
> skilled touch, patient watchfulness and unwearied vigils,
> are as great factors in the care of the sick, as are
> the professional physicians."
>
> — Lydia Hoyt Farmer

Why did you become a nurse? Was it because you wanted to spend long hours on your feet and under stress? Perhaps it was because you enjoy working with cranky patients and condescending doctors.

Or was it because nursing gave you a chance to make a difference?

Do you ever wonder what your patients think of you when you leave their rooms or they check out?

Even if sometimes it doesn't seem that you're making a difference, or even appreciated, you can rest assured that your patients know who you are and that you're working for their benefit. And you do make a difference in our lives every moment that you spend with us.

It takes an extremely special person to pursue a nursing career. Nurses must be nurturing yet strong, sensible yet caring and, above all else, selfless as they go about their vital duties.

At times, the job may seem thankless. Ongoing demands from patients and medical staff alike can deflate even the most hard-working spirit. But determined nurses embrace their role despite long hours and aching feet.

Yes, patients have high expectations for you, and sometimes, yes, those expectations are unreasonable. But more often than not, you exceed our expectations, although we may not realize it until later.

Why do we have these expectations, and why are we sometimes dissatisfied despite your best efforts? Most of the time, it's because we don't know what we need from you, or even what we want other than to get better. Mostly, you see us when our bodies are sick or broken. At those times, we are plunged into a new world that frightens us, that we don't understand. When we're sick, we lose control of all or a part of our lives, and it seems to us that that control passes into the hands of you and our doctors.

Here are some of our expectations and how you fulfill them.

We believe that you have knowledge of our bodies that we will never have, and that you know how to apply that knowledge in a way that helps us get better. You teach us and reassure us that this is the case. Thank you.

We believe that you want us to get better and will do all you can to make

> "Nurses are angels in comfortable shoes."
>
> — Author Unknown

6

it happen. You give us a word or a touch that says, "Yes, I can help you. I will help you." Thank you.

We believe that you really want to know us as people, not simply names on a schedule, or documentation on a chart. Sometimes you take five minutes to ask about our lives beyond our medical conditions. Thank you.

We believe that you are thinking and caring about us even when you are not with us. You surprise us with a book or magazine that we mentioned in passing, or a postcard with a picture of a place we said was a favorite. Thank you.

Yes, we believe that you _are_ very special. But how often do you show us how special you really are? Most of your job is hidden from us. You consult a chart, you look at a machine, you listen to our hearts, you adjust an IV — what do you see or hear? We want to know about these things. We want to appreciate your knowledge and your heart.

This book was written to let you know how remarkable we think you are, and what you can do to help us appreciate your knowledge and skill. As patients in bad situations, we need nurses to share much more to ease both our pain and our minds. We rely on nurses for comfort, exceptional care and expertise.

ANN'S STORY

Part I

I will always remember the day I first saw you. I was jogging at City Park when suddenly I felt very tired — my breath turned to gasps and my heart pounded. I'd had episodes of sudden fatigue like this many times before, but this time my legs began to strain so hard they actually ached. The muscles in my hips felt like they were on fire. I felt like I was running through molasses. My body wanted to stop — and it did.

The next thing I remember was the ambulance. My throat was dry, and my tongue felt swollen. There was an oxygen mask over my mouth and nose. A paramedic sat over me, talking into his radio. "Female, approximately 38, unconscious, no external injuries, B/P 110 over 60."

I remember thinking, "Is it a bad sign when the EMS guy says you look four years older than your actual age?" The paramedic looked down at me and saw my eyes were open. "Oh, hey! Hi there! You're going to be okay." I tried to say "hi" back — I'm not sure if I did. He took my pulse and wrote it down. Then he looked at me and asked, "We're on our way to the hospital. Do you have insurance?" I nodded.

Hospital! The word fluttered up in front of my eyes. My senses were suddenly overwhelmed — the cold fluorescent light, the prickly smell of antiseptic, the atmosphere of dread, people who ask you about your insurance before they know your name. Then I was very tired again. A wave of fatigue swept up from my feet. I tried to tell the paramedic, "I'm going to sleep now." And I did.

The next time I opened my eyes, I was looking up at a high ceiling and into the glare of cold fluorescent lights. The tang of antiseptic was in my nostrils. Hospital! My heart sank. And then, there you were — your smiling face cutting through the glare of the lights. "Well, hello there," you said. "You have such pretty eyes — it's nice to finally see them open."

(to be continued)

1

THE BASICS

"The needs of a human being are sacred. Their satisfaction cannot be subordinated either to reasons of state, or to any consideration of money, nationality, race, or color, or to the moral or other value attributed to the human being in question, or to any consideration whatsoever."

— Simone Weil

We all share basic needs. Air, fluids, food, sleep, waste elimination, shelter, and security are at the top. Sometimes we have trouble meeting one or more of those needs — we need help. This is particularly true when we are injured or ill.

Some of us enjoy having someone like you to help us out, but many of us are uncomfortable receiving help from anyone. Because the basic needs are so fundamental to our existence, relying on someone else to provide them requires trust, and trust is not something most of us easily invest in people we don't know. It may adversely affect the way we respond to even the kindest of your gestures. In spite of what we may say or do, we know that we need your help, and we always appreciate it.

> "Our needs hourly
> Climb and return like angels.
> Unclosing like a hand,
> You give forever."
> — Philip Larkin

We know you do a fantastic job monitoring our vital signs and watching for the more visible signs of distress such as low oxygen levels, pallor or hyperventilation.

We think you're amazing when you see the things that aren't as obvious. For example, when we're anxious or worried, we may not be able to get the sleep we need for our bodies to mend. When you notice we're not sleeping, your reassurance and comfort help us relax. If we still have trouble sleeping, a quick word to a doctor on our behalf may cause an alteration or addition to our treatment that alleviates the problem. Knowing that you are paying attention and seeing you making efforts to get us the things we need builds our trust. When you acknowledge our needs and let us know you are taking action to meet those needs, our fear decreases and our confidence rises. Thank you.

Basic needs are often difficult to ask for. Sometimes we don't think you can do something that you really can do, like help us get a quieter room. Sometimes we're just uncomfortable with the nature of the need. Bedpans and wet sheets are everyday things for you, but asking for a bedpan or change of sheets may be very painful for us psychologically. We may even ask for something different from what we really need. For example, we may ask for food or water, when what we really want is company and comfort.

You can't imagine how much it means to us when you take that extra moment to soothe our fears and let us know it's okay to ask for whatever we need.

Sometimes we feel much worse than we really are; other times we feel much better than we really are. It's often difficult to accurately assess our own true conditions. We rely on you to help us with that. When you let us know what to expect and explain what's really going on, it makes us feel more secure. When we understand more about our situations, we're better able to focus on doing the things we need to do to get well.

We know we try your patience when we do things or want to do things that are not good for us. For example, we may not be able to eat or drink because of tests or surgery. Or we may need to be on a special, not-so-appetizing-diet for a while. When the restrictions seem arbitrary, we may be tempted to sneak forbidden items. It's our way of trying to take back some control. When you explain the reasons for restrictions and how they can help us get better, our efforts at regaining control can be directed toward taking more responsibility for our own care and recovery.

"Patience serves as a protection against wrongs as clothes do against cold. For if you put on more clothes as the cold increases, it will have no power to hurt you. So in like manner you must grow in patience when you meet with great wrongs, and they will then be powerless to vex your mind."
— Leonardo da Vinci

Our basic needs are sometimes overlooked or taken for granted. When we see you making positive efforts to provide these needs even in difficult circumstances, we think you are incredible. You truly do make a difference. Thank you.

ANN'S STORY

Part 2

I felt like I had the worst hangover ever. My body ached, my head ached, my brain was full of fog, and my mouth dry and sticky. "Is this the hospital?" I rasped.

"The emergency room," you said, nodding.

"What happened to me?"

"Well, that's what we're wondering. Your vital signs are all good, and you don't appear to be wounded. We were hoping you could help us out a little. Do you feel like talking?"

"Could I have some water?" I asked.

"Sure. Do you think you can sit up?"

"I think so."

You adjusted the bed so I could sit up.

"Ow!" I suddenly got a sharp pain in my belly.

"What? What happened?" You took my hand and looked into my eyes with concern.

"I don't know … a pain … here. It's okay, it's going away."

You probed gently around my abdomen. "Any more pain? Here? Or here?"

"No. It's okay."

"Still feel like that water?"

"Yes, please," I said gratefully. You handed me the glass and I drank, soothing my raw throat.

(to be continued)

2

SECURITY AND SAFETY

"In a multitude of acquaintances is less security,
than in one faithful friend."
— Herman Melville

Security and safety are almost as important to us as our physiological needs — in some cases, more so. After all, having access to food, water and shelter doesn't mean much if we live in constant dread of having them taken away, or our lives are threatened. Letting us know that we are secure and safe early on is a good way to establish a relationship with us that will shorten our time in your care and make your job easier.

Of course, safety and security can mean different things to us. To some of us it may be something as simple as a hug at an appropriate moment. To others, it could be a prayer, and still others, the knowledge and trust that someone will be there when we need help. When you understand what we, as individuals, need to feel secure and safe and make the effort to give us those things, you give us the wonderful gift of peace of mind. Thank you.

Safety and security are first and foremost about communication. Your experience and knowledge gives you special insight into the needs of patients in our situations. When you use this understanding to communicate with us both verbally and non-verbally, your stature automatically rises in our eyes — your professional status is confirmed and puts us at ease.

To us, medicine today often appears to be all about machines and drugs. It seems the responsibility for our recoveries depends on chemicals with names we can't pronounce and machines that look like they should be on the space shuttle. But you know that's not all there is to care and healing.

As you go about your routine tasks and let us know what you're doing and why you're doing it, we feel a greater sense of individuality and become more involved in our own recoveries. When you insert IVs into our veins or paste sensors to monitoring machines on our skin and you explain what's going into our bodies and why we need it, and that the scary-looking boxes next to our beds help you keep tabs on our conditions and alert you if something needs attention, we begin to see those things that seemed impersonal and forbidding as ways to provide us with greater security and safety.

Maintaining our privacy is another way we can feel more secure. When you do something as simple as making sure a door is closed or a curtain drawn when we're undressed or being examined, we feel that you care about preserving our dignity and see us as more than just "cases" to be processed. Privacy can also be more than just physical. We trust that you won't discuss our conditions with people who don't need to know, or do so in a place or at a volume where outsiders can hear. We rest assured knowing that you realize this can destroy our sense of security and break the bonds of trust you work so hard to nurture.

> "Nothing is quite as bad as being without privacy and lonely at the same time."
> — Alexander Theroux

Did you know we also feel safer and more secure when we have a routine we can count on? Providing at least a modicum of structure for us lets us know what to expect from you and when to expect it. We feel more in control when we know, even in small ways, what's in store for us. Having difficult ongoing treatments or exams at about the same times each day allows us to prepare mentally and physically for the challenges.

We look forward to the times when you come by to check on us. Knowing that we can expect you to stop by with a story or a joke or a word of comfort gives us the confidence that we are safe and not forgotten. Our spirits are lifted when we know when we can expect visitors. Conversely, if we are tired or not feeling well, we also appreciate you when you come by to shoo visitors out promptly at the end of visiting hours. Thank you.

Your sensitivity to the environment around us and confidently taking action to change things when our reactions are adverse, or reinforcing positive responses relieves our fears and gives us the confidence to relax and face whatever is in store for us with the mind-set that all will be well. When you ensure that we have positive relationships with our environments, it enhances our relationships with you, and gives us the power and desire to cooperate and help you to do your best.

ANN'S STORY

Part 3
"You were in running clothes when the EMTs brought you in. Is that what you were doing when you fainted?"

I nodded, fingering the flimsy gown in which I was now draped, and told you about the unfamiliar muscle aches I'd begun to get while running a few weeks before and that I figured it was just my age catching up with me. I also told you about my pooping out sooner than I had in the past, and once again used the age excuse. You smiled and made notes, and then went on to take the rest of my history. Your warmth and concern, and the way you asked your questions made me feel like I was talking to an old friend rather than an emergency room nurse. We even had a little discussion about my collection of glass figurines.

The doctor came in a few minutes later and checked me. She asked about stress (a little more than usual at work), my eating habits (no changes), and sleep (sleeping very well). She looked at me — puzzled, it seemed to me — then went out and talked to you for a few moments.

You came in smiling and said, "Well, the good news is, it doesn't seem to be anything serious. The bad news is, you seem quite healthy, so we don't really know why you fainted. The doctor would like to keep you overnight for observation. She isn't making it mandatory, but it would be a good idea."

"Observation. What does that mean exactly?" I asked, not liking the sound of it.

"Nothing sinister," you laughed. "You just spend the night and we check on you every now and then, and see if something happens. To be honest, most of the time, nothing does. You'll wake up in the morning, a doctor will take another look at you, and then you'll get dressed and go home."

I sighed, "Okay, you convinced me. But could I ask you a favor?"

"Sure."

"I prefer to go running on an empty stomach, so I haven't had anything to eat since this morning. Is there a vending machine or somewhere I could get a snack?"

"They'll be serving dinner around the time we get you checked in, but I'll see if I can rustle up something for you to take the edge off."

(to be continued)

3

CARING AND BELONGING

> "Kindness makes the difference between passion and caring. Kindness is tenderness. Kindness is love, but perhaps greater than love. Kindness is good will. Kindness says, 'I want you to be happy.' Kindness comes very close to the benevolence of God."
> — Randolph Ray

All people need interaction with other people — isolation and exile are punishments in every human society. When we are ill or injured, we especially need to feel a sense of belonging and have people who care about us. The stress of pain or discomfort and being removed from our normal surroundings can make us feel disconnected, lost. The comfort of a kind voice and a gentle touch can relieve at least some of that stress.

Even when we have the support of loved ones, when we feel we can count on you as a medical professional to be part of that support group, we become charged with the power we need to fight the disease or heal the injury.

Unfortunately, some of us don't have friends or family to support us — in these cases, you and your colleagues are our support group. With so many families becoming disconnected as they move away for job opportunities, this is a common, lonely reality for many. There is nothing worse than being single in a city without family to offer unconditional love, a hand to hold or a ready hug. We rely more and more on others to fill this role. Without you, an examining room or a hospital room can be a very lonely place.

A hospital or medical office is by necessity cold and sterile, but a messy sort of warmth is fundamental to our connection with others and our well-being. We don't expect hugs every time you check on us, but just remembering our names and using them can spark immediate connections with us. And telling us your name completes the circuit. We know each other now. You're not just an anonymous functionary in scrubs — you're our nurse!

Some of us come to you because we've caused ourselves or found ourselves in trouble. But you are a professional caregiver and you treat us with patience and respect. We may be judged and rejected by the outside world, but when we're in your care, we belong to a very special group — your patients. We cherish that connection and return the respect. Thank you.

Lighting up our rooms with your smile, and reassuring us with your eye contact are the simple things you do to bring a positive response. They also help you to assess our conditions. You know this kind of contact makes you more open to our feelings. You know enough about us to start conversations that can give you helpful insights into our conditions. Your soft touch, your gentle squeeze of the hand lessens our tension and makes us more responsive to your instructions. Your calm, soothing demeanor, even when you're trying to resolve serious problems, gives us confidence.

We know that you care about us and want us to get better. Others may see us as lab reports, or blood-pressure readings, but you see us as valuable and necessary parts of your world. And we feel like valued members of your family.

"By building relations, we create a source of love and personal pride and belonging that makes living in a chaotic world easier."
— Susan Lieberman

ANN'S STORY

Part 4

A few minutes later you returned with a bag containing two bran muffins. "From my lunch," you said. "You can thank a kid with a broken arm who came in before I could get to them."

"Homemade?" I asked.

"Sure," you laughed, "of course, it was Betty Crocker's home, but I did get to use my mixer."

You left and I happily downed your muffins. With my hunger eased, you returned and began helping me with the paperwork to check into the hospital. A few minutes later I was doubled over again with sharp pains in my belly.

You looked stricken, "Oh my God, it's the muffins!"

"No, no," I gasped. "This is the same as before!"

You ran out to get the doctor. A couple of minutes later you were back with her, but the pain was already subsiding. "You're checking in, aren't you?" the doctor asked. I nodded. "Good, we definitely want to keep an eye on you tonight. Have you had pains like this before?" she asked, probing my belly and around my face and neck.

"Yes, not too often. Usually after eating. It's mostly just gas."

"Have you ever been diagnosed with fibromyalgia?" the doctor asked.

"What?" I said, my eyes growing wide.

"Fibromyalgia," she repeated.

"No! Why? Is that what I have?"

The doctor made some notes and said, "It's a possibility. Let's get you settled in upstairs and then we'll see." She turned and left the cubicle.

I anxiously looked to you for help, "What is that … fibromy…?"

You smiled reassuringly, "It's a condition that has some of your symptoms."

"Is it serious?"

"Well, yes, it can be, but she's just making a guess. There are a lot of other things it could be, too. We'll have to do some tests to find out for sure. Here, let's finish these forms and get you into a room."

(to be continued)

4

ESTEEM

> "Self-esteem creates natural highs. Knowing that you're lovable helps you to love more. Knowing that you're important helps you to make a difference to others. Knowing that you are capable empowers you to create more. Knowing that you're valuable and that you have a special place in the universe is a serene spiritual joy in itself."
>
> — Louise Hart

We all need a sense of self-respect and self-esteem. We also need to have respect for others and have others respect us. When we lack self-esteem, we tend to draw into ourselves and become disengaged from our communities. Disengagement makes it difficult for us to do the things that allow others to recognize and respect us, which can cause our self-esteem to sink even further. Our self-esteem often suffers when we are ill, and low self-esteem can cause problems with our recoveries — feelings of helplessness and worthlessness are not attitudes that support our immune and healing systems.

Many of us feel guilty about being sick and causing trouble for our families or friends. You give our self-esteem a boost when you reassure us that illness and accidents are a part of everyone's lives, and that we will all need help at some point. In fact, these are times, even opportunities, to learn more about ourselves and deepen our relationships with others. You reassure us when you help us make a smooth transition to patient status. You let us know that it's okay for us to give up some control and let others care for us for a time. You show regard for our dignity and respect our individuality despite our temporary dependence. Thank you.

An important aspect of building self-esteem in others is maintaining your own self-esteem. We respect and admire all nurses' dedication to and skill in caring for others, and we gain confidence when you display pride and confidence in your professionalism. You understand yourself and your reasons for becoming a nurse, and this allows you to understand us and help us better cope with our conditions.

Your fresh, professional appearance displays your pride and self-esteem for all to see. We admire the way you keep yourself physically fit and manage the stress that we all know comes with your job. When you are off the job, you concentrate on caring for yourself and your family. You do things you love to do, whether it be going on a hike, reading a book, gardening, or having a picnic with your family. Your interesting life away from the job not only relieves your stress, it makes you an interesting person, someone we want to know and with whom we can build a productive relationship that benefits us all.

Positive self-esteem feeds off itself. It opens us up to new experiences. It makes us more interesting *to* others, and more interested *in* others. The foundations of our society are built on this kind of reciprocal engagement. When we are injured or ill, it makes us look forward to returning to our lives, healthy and well. We want to work with you and cooperate in our treatment so we can get better as quickly as possible.

ANN'S STORY

Part 5

A half-hour later, I was in a pale-green, sterile room. I was cold enough to be under a blanket — alone, and worried.

An orderly showed up a few minutes later with a cart full of dinner trays. He set me up with the bed table and plunked a tray on it. There was steamed chicken breast, noodles with some kind of white sauce, a biscuit, a brownie, and a glass of red liquid. None of it looked particularly appetizing, but I was ravenous and I went at it with determination if not gusto.

About halfway through the meal, you knocked and came in. You were off-duty and could have been home with your family, but there you were, and my glum mood instantly turned around.

"I just wanted to see if you got settled in okay," you said. "And I brought you a little something."

You handed me a small box. I opened it and inside was a beautiful little glass unicorn. I was speechless.

"It was in the gift shop. I thought it might make the room a little less forbidding for you," you said.

"Oh yes! Thank you! Thank you so much. I love it. You didn't have to…."

"I know, I know, but I know how it feels being rushed into a strange place, not knowing what's going to happen. So you got dinner? How does it taste?"

"Well, it doesn't really have much of a taste."

"Good, that's the way it's supposed to be. If a chef makes something that tastes good, she's immediately fired," you said, laughing.

I laughed with you, and suddenly the pain returned to my belly, sharp and intense. I doubled forward, knocking over the glass of red liquid. You jumped up.

"Are you okay? Is it the same thing?"

"Yes," I gasped. "What is that?" The pain remained, but the sharpness faded, and I lay back onto the pillows. You grabbed a towel from the bathroom and cleaned up around the bed, pushing the table with the nearly finished meal away.

"I'm going to get the doctor and the nurse, I'll be right back," you said, heading for the door.

Suddenly I sat upright again, "No, no, wait! The bathroom! I need … I need … the bathroom!

You rushed back and helped me to the bathroom. The diarrhea was so intense I wouldn't have made it without your help. You got me settled on the toilet and then ran out again to get the doctor and nurse.

A little while later, I was back in bed with clean sheets and the resident poking at my body. You stood by the door smiling.

The resident made some notes and looked at me, "Well, everything seems to be back in order. The night nurse will keep an eye on you tonight, and in the morning we'll run a few tests and get to the bottom of this. Okay?" He patted my hand.

"Okay," I said.

The resident went into the corridor. You followed and stopped him. You spoke with him for a minute — I couldn't hear, but it was clearly about me. The resident nodded, made another note, and left.

Then you came back in and introduced me to the night nurse, "She's a good friend and a good nurse. She'll take care of you," you said. "You'll be fine, don't worry."

My belief in you was complete. "I know," I said. "I don't know how to thank you."

"Hey, I'm a nurse. It's what we do, right?" you said, laughing. You gave me a hug, and then you were gone.

I looked to the side table for my unicorn. Its horn had gotten broken in the scuffling, but it didn't matter. I held it in my hands and eventually fell asleep.

(to be continued)

5

SELF-EXPRESSION AND KNOWLEDGE

"Knowledge is indivisible. When people grow wise in one direction, they are sure to make it easier for themselves to grow wise in other directions as well. On the other hand, when they split up knowledge, concentrate on their own field, and scorn and ignore other fields, they grow less wise — even in their own field."

— Isaac Asimov

All of us have a limited time in this life, and all of us have a need to make the most of that time. The essence of being human is carrying on and moving forward, making the attempt to become better people today than we were yesterday. Illness and injury can sap our energy, stop our forward momentum, and cause us to substitute complaint and judgment toward others for fruitful self-expression and learning.

When we show an interest in pursuing self-expression and knowledge, we generally have, or are on our way to, good physical and mental health. When you pay attention to our level of interest in things outside ourselves, you have a pretty good indicator of how we are progressing in our treatments and recoveries. When you try to stimulate these interests in us, you show us that you are thinking of us beyond our charts and readings. You remind us that we aren't defined by our sickness. You let us know that we are worthwhile and that overcoming our illness matters. Thank you.

> "There are thousands of causes for stress, and one antidote to stress is self-expression."
> — Garson Kanin

A good way to stimulate self-expression and knowledge is to communicate with us. Do we understand what's going on, what's going to happen and why you're doing what you're doing? We all naturally have questions. You make us feel comfortable asking them, and you answer them to the best of your ability. Just asking how we feel, and helping us to understand why we feel the way we do, moves us outside of ourselves and helps us see our conditions objectively and rationally. Because you listen to us and take good notes, you remember our conversations the next time you see us. This helps give us a sense that our treatment has continuity and is moving forward.

You are the expert and we look to you to provide helpful and practical information. When we're ill, or even just nervous, we don't always remember what we're told. You are patient with us and provide us with reminders. You give explanations as many times as necessary for us to understand.

Doctors often say things we don't understand, and we are often intimidated by doctors. You never assume that we really understand, even when we tell the doctor we do. You give us explanations suitable for our levels of understanding. You reassure us that the doctor's use of elaborate medical jargon doesn't indicate the severity of our conditions, and you put complicated concepts in plain words so we can grasp them.

Sometimes doctors *don't* say things that we are expecting them to say. When we're worried and unsure, no news is not always good news. You see to it that we get any information we feel is missing. Thank you.

We are grateful when you act as our representative with the doctors. We frequently want to explain our feelings to our doctors, but sometimes it's hard to put those feelings into words, and we don't want to waste their time. You have spent time with us and listened to us. You understand us even when we're not sure how to say the things we need to say. Effective communication is key to medical treatment, and sometimes we need an interpreter. Thank you for translating.

You feed our inherent quest for knowledge when you educate us about our conditions and our surroundings. We are naturally fearful of things we don't understand. Our control is threatened. Our fates don't seem to be in our hands. When you talk with us about our illnesses or injuries, the procedures and treatments, and the tools you use, you satisfy our

"The secret of joy in work is contained in one word — excellence. To know how to do something well is to enjoy it."

— Pearl Buck

natural curiosity and help return a sense of control to us. We are most appreciative when you let us know what to expect. Imagine how much easier it is for us when, for example, *prior to surgery and before the pain starts*, you explain about the importance of post-surgical oxygenation and how to practice deep

> "It takes a long time to bring excellence to maturity."
> — Publilius Syrus

breathing to speed healing. You help us understand what to expect and what we can do to help ourselves.

Above all, we rely on you to be honest and truthful. We can all remember occasions when people have lied to us or shaded the truth, not maliciously, but "for our own good." Do we ever really trust these people again? We know you guard your integrity as if it was your most precious possession, because you know it is.

One of the best things you do is admit when you're wrong, or simply don't know. We understand mistakes — we all make them. We understand not having all the information we need immediately at hand. You build our confidence when, after giving us wrong information, you come back to us, admit your mistake, and then give us the correct information. When we ask you a question and you're not sure of the answer, you don't guess, you tell us you will find the correct answer, and then do it. For that honesty, our opinions of you are not lessened, they soar, along with our sense of security.

And we expect that you will pay attention to your own needs for self-expression and knowledge. We know that medical techniques and practice are continually evolving, and we know that you take pains to keep yourself up to date and bring that new knowledge to the workplace with you. We know that you regard us as resources for your expansion of knowledge. We think you are so lucky to have the opportunity to interact with such a variety of people at such an intimate level. As you are generous with the sharing of your knowledge, we will be generous with our knowledge. Many of the most ordinary-looking of us have had extraordinary lives — often, all it takes to open these troves to your view are a couple of simple questions.

Building relationships that feed all our needs for self-expression and knowledge helps us in our recoveries, increases your professional skills and provides us all with feelings of accomplishment and satisfaction. This is the way you make a difference to us that we can cherish throughout our lives.

ANN'S STORY

Part 6

The next day, I had several tests done, including the one that you suggested to the resident the evening before. That was the one that came up positive, and I had a name for my illness — Celiac disease, gluten-intolerance. It wasn't the most welcome news I could have gotten, but I have it under control now, and I'm doing fine. I found out later that it's a very difficult disease to diagnose. The resident told me that if you hadn't made your suggestion, we might not have figured it out for weeks. How did you know?

I never saw you again. You were off duty that next day. I could have gone back to the ER later and found you, but I didn't want to bother you. And I don't really need to see you — every time I glance at my shelves of glass figurines, I see the unicorn with the broken horn right up front, and I imagine you coming into other people's lives and performing your incredible magic. Thank you.

6

The Extra Step

> "Beauty is no quality in things themselves:
> It exists merely in the mind which contemplates them;
> and each mind perceives a different beauty."
> — David Hume

D o you remember the last time you had a bad case of the flu? With your aches and pains and fevers, did you care that there were dirty dishes in the sink, or the garbage can was full? Did you grab the vacuum when you noticed a dust ball under the dresser? Did you put on fresh clothes every day or just thrash about in the same sweaty pajamas? Was a daily bath high on your priority list?

There's nothing like sickness to turn the most immaculate of us into slobs. It's not that we don't want to be fresh and clean, or look our best, and it's not that we lose our appreciation of our surroundings. We simply have more important things to do. In sickness, it's our job to heal ourselves. But there is no doubt that the aesthetic aspects of our environments have effects on our health. A NASCAR poster can remind a disheartened racing fan of good times he's had at the track

"Beauty can be feasted on."
— Chinese proverb

and make him look forward to a full recovery and more good times with family and friends. A vase of chrysanthemums can bring a little bit of the natural beauty a depressed gardener misses so much into her room and lift her spirits. **The simplest of things, like helping us into a change of clothes, or combing our hair, or supporting us so we can brush our teeth, gives us a morale boost that cannot be measured. Thank you.**

We understand that the demands on your time and energy are overwhelming. We understand that checking and recording our vital signs comes first. We understand that making sure we have the correct dosages of the correct medications and seeing that the doctors have all the supplies and tools they need to do their jobs are your priorities. We understand that cleansing wounds and administering life-saving emergency procedures are vastly more important than our makeup or a spot of color in our gray rooms. But when you make that extra effort, even with the smallest of gestures, you remind us of the beauty in our lives and make us all the more anxious to get back to it. You make a difference, and we will never forget you.

Some Good Reasons to Be a Nurse

♦ Nurses are in demand.

♦ The pay is good and getting better.

♦ You can work almost anywhere you want.

♦ You can work almost any time you want.

♦ You have job security.

♦ The job is open to anyone possessing passion and dedication.

♦ There are many different areas and specialties from which to choose.

♦ If you feel you are becoming burned out, you can easily change to a different type of nursing.

♦ Nurses are respected for their knowledge and their caring natures.

♦ It's a job that makes a difference.

Thank you, Nurse!

"I can testify that friendship has literally cured a fever, and the medicine of daily affection, a bad wound. In these sayings are the final secret of carrying out well the role of an hospital missionary."
— Walt Whitman

ABOUT THE AUTHOR

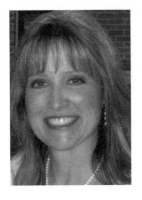

Debbie Phillips, R.N.

Debbie grew up in Southern California and moved to Texas after receiving a degree in Registered Nursing in 1981. She has worked for over 26 years as an office nurse and surgical first assistant. This has given her the opportunity to build relationships with patients and follow them throughout their care while keeping in touch with her nursing skills.

She has been fortunate to work for two very successful surgeons who have promoted her growth and responsibilities. Debbie has done everything from ordering supplies, scheduling, pre-operative workups, post-operative care, patient education and dressing changes — to name just a few!

Debbie has organized and taught classes for patient education programs on Woman's Health Issues and Surgical Procedures at local hospitals. She has also been on six medical missions to El Salvador as a participant with Austin Smiles, a nonprofit organization that organizes medical teams to provide no-charge corrective surgeries for children with cleft lips and palates.

Debbie continues to be passionate about her career and is looking forward to the different adventures that nursing offers.

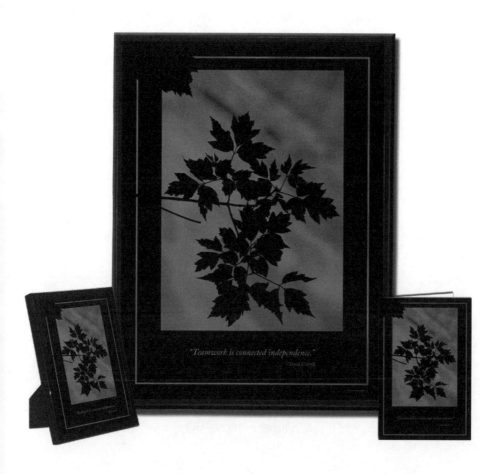

Accelerate Personal Growth Resources

12 Choices…That Lead to Your Success is about success…how to achieve it, keep it and enjoy it…by making better choices. $14.95

Orchestrating Attitude translates the incomprehensible into the actionable. It cuts through the clutter to deliver inspiration and application so you can orchestrate your attitude…and your success. $9.95

Conquering Adversity – Six Strategies to Move You and Your Team Through Tough Times is a practical guide to help people and organizations deal with the unexpected and move forward through adversity. $14.95

107 Ways to Stick to It What's the REAL secret to success? Learn the secrets from the world's highest achievers. These 107 practical, inspiring tips will help you stick to it and WIN! $9.95

The Ant and the Elephant is a different kind of book for a different kind of leader! A great story that teaches that we must lead ourselves before we can expect to be an effective leader of others. $12.95

Too Many Emails contains dozens of tips and techniques to increase your email effectiveness and efficiency. $9.95

175 Ways to Get More Done in Less Time has 175 really good suggestions that will help you get things done faster…usually better. $9.95

Becoming the Obvious Choice is a roadmap showing each employee how they can maintain their motivation, develop their hidden talents and become the best. $9.95

You and Your Network is profitable reading for those who want to learn how to develop healthy relationships with others. "I think every living person should read and re-read this book. It can change your life." – David Cottrell $9.95

136 Effective Presentation Tips is a powerful handbook providing 136 practical, easy to use tips to make every presentation a success. $9.95

Silver Bullets contains straightforward tips on how to gain success while keeping your wits about you. $14.95

The NEW CornerStone Perpetual Calendar, a compelling collection of quotes about leadership and life, is perfect for office desks, school and home countertops. $14.95

CornerStone Collection of Note Cards Sampler Pack is designed to make it easy for you to show appreciation for your team, clients and friends. The awesome photography and your personal message written inside will create a lasting impact. Pack of 12 (one each of all 12 designs) $24.95

Visit www.**CornerStoneLeadership**.com for additional books and resources.

YES! Please send me extra copies of *Thank You, Nurse!*
1-99 copies $9.95   100-999 copies $8.95   1000+ copies $7.95

Thank You, Nurse!	_____ copies X _____	= $ _____

Additional Personal Growth Resources

Accelerate Personal Growth Package   _____ pack(s) X $139.95   = $ _____
(Includes one each of all items listed
on page 46.)

Other Books

	_____ copies X _____	= $ _____
_____	_____ copies X _____	= $ _____
_____	_____ copies X _____	= $ _____
_____	_____ copies X _____	= $ _____
_____	_____ copies X _____	= $ _____
	Shipping & Handling	$ _____
	Subtotal	$ _____
	Sales Tax (8.25%-TX Only)	$ _____
	Total (U.S. Dollars Only)	$ _____

Shipping and Handling Charges

Total $ Amount	Up to $49	$50-$99	$100-$249	$250-$1199	$1200-$2999	$3000+
Charge	$6	$9	$16	$30	$80	$125

Name _____ Job Title _____

Organization _____ Phone_____

Shipping Address _____ Fax _____

Billing Address _____ E-mail _____
(required when ordering PowerPoint® Presentation)

City _____ State _____ ZIP_____

❑ Please invoice (Orders over $200) Purchase Order Number (if applicable)   _____

Charge Your Order: ❑ MasterCard   ❑ Visa   ❑ American Express

Credit Card Number _____ Exp. Date _____

Signature _____

❑ Check Enclosed (Payable to: CornerStone Leadership)

Fax	**Mail**	**Phone**
972.274.2884	**P.O. Box 764087**	**888.789.5323**
	Dallas, TX 75376	

www.**CornerStoneLeadership**.com

Thank you for reading *Thank You, Nurse!*
We hope it has assisted you in your quest for
personal and professional growth.

CornerStone Leadership is committed to provide new
and enlightening products to organizations worldwide.
Our mission is to fuel knowledge with practical resources
that will accelerate your team's productivity,
success and job satisfaction!

Best wishes for your continued success.

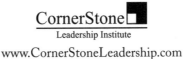

CornerStone
Leadership Institute
www.CornerStoneLeadership.com

*Start a crusade in your organization –
have the courage to learn, the vision to lead,
and the passion to share.*